Finding Purpose in the Storm

Darius Marshall

DEDICATION

Dedicated to his two resilient daughters P & F, this book is a testament to the strength, courage, and perseverance they have shown in the face of adversity. Through this dedication, the author honors the extraordinary resilience and tenacity displayed by his daughters, acknowledging the challenges they have overcome with grace and determination.

In a heartfelt show of appreciation, the author expresses deep gratitude to the staff at the IWK for their attentive care, support, and compassion towards his daughter. This acknowledgment serves as a tribute to the dedicated professionals who listened, empathized, and provided invaluable assistance during a challenging time.

Acknowledging Donna's warm and cheerful presence during their hospital stay, the author expresses heartfelt gratitude for her kindness and thoughtfulness. By recognizing Donna's efforts in making their time at the hospital enjoyable through her smiles and gestures like providing ice cream, the author highlights the significance of small acts of kindness in brightening difficult moments.

SARAH'S STORY

Sarah skipped through the park, her golden curls bouncing in the sunlight, a trail of giggles left in her wake. The vibrant hues of blooming flowers painted a picturesque backdrop to her carefree dance, as she joyfully chased after butterflies, her laughter a melodic symphony that echoed through the air.

In the warmth of her family's love, Sarah's days were a patchwork of joy and contentment. Her parents' comforting embrace was a sanctuary where worries melted away, and the world felt like a safe, welcoming place. Days were spent exploring nature's wonders, picnicking under the shade of ancient trees, and sharing stories that wove the fabric of their tightly knit family even closer.

Yet, as Sarah's innocent laughter filled the air, a subtle shift began to stir beneath the surface of her idyllic existence. It started as a faint tweet—a barely perceptible sound, a fleeting tic that danced across her face. At first, her family dismissed it as harmless quirks of childhood, attributing them to innocent whims and passing fancies.

But as days turned into weeks, the bird tweets grew more pronounced, evolving into tics that seemed to have a life of their own. The once carefree skip in her step faltered at times, her jovial laughter tinged with a hint of uncertainty. Sarah's family watched with growing concern, their brows furrowed with worry as they tried to unravel the mystery behind these unexpected changes.

Despite the undercurrent of unease that began to thread its way through their lives, Sarah's family enveloped her in a bubble of love and understanding, determined to weather whatever storm lay ahead. Little did they know that these seemingly insignificant tremors were the faint whispers of a greater challenge—one that would test not only Sarah's resilience but also the very fabric of their unbreakable bond.

As Sarah continued to navigate her daily routines, the once faint tremors that had initially unsettled her family began to morph into more pronounced manifestations. What had started as subtle audible tics—a soft clearing of her throat, a gentle hum that escaped her lips—began to evolve into uncontrollable physical twitches and jerks that seemed to have a life of their own.

During her morning walks in the park, Sarah's skipping gait turned erratic, interrupted by sudden, involuntary movements that caused her to stumble. Her laughter, once a constant melody in the air, now mingled with the sound of sporadic grunts and sniffles that she couldn't suppress. The butterflies she had once joyfully chased now fluttered around her in a chaotic dance, mirroring the inner turmoil she tried so hard to conceal.

At home, the safety of her family's comforting embrace became a battleground of conflicting emotions. Her parents watched with aching hearts as their vibrant, carefree daughter struggled to contain the physical tics that seemed to have taken hold of her once nimble limbs. The worried glances they exchanged spoke volumes, silent prayers whispered for a return to the simplicity of days gone by.

Sarah, too, grappled with a storm of emotions within. The once confident child found herself shrinking under the weight of her body's betrayals, her sunny disposition clouded by a sense of helplessness and confusion. The mirror reflected a distorted image of herself—one she barely recognized—a girl caught in the throes of a battle she had never anticipated.

Despite the challenges that loomed on the horizon, a flicker of determination stirred within Sarah's soul. With each passing day, she drew strength from the unwavering support of her family, clinging to the hope that amidst the chaos of her unraveling world, there lay a path to acceptance, resilience, and the unwavering belief that she was more than the sum of her tics.

As Sarah's physical tics escalated, a new layer of complexity began to weave itself into the fabric of her reality. Alongside the involuntary movements and audible outbursts, dark hallucinations crept into her world like shadowy specters, casting a sinister pall over the once vibrant landscape of her mind.

During her walks in the park, the whispering winds seemed to carry eerie voices that beckoned her towards unseen depths. The trees that once stood tall and majestic now morphed into twisted, menacing shapes that seemed to reach out towards her with gnarled branches, their leaves rustling with a malevolent intent that sent shivers down her spine.

As she chased after butterflies, their delicate wings transformed into grotesque, shifting shapes that taunted her with twisted messages that only she could hear. The laughter that once echoed through the air now mingled with chilling cries and haunting whispers that seemed to seep into her very being, leaving her trembling with a mixture of fear and confusion.

At home, the once familiar walls of her sanctuary seemed to warp and distort, their surfaces pulsating with dark, swirling patterns that danced before her eyes like a macabre symphony. Shadows lurked in every corner, their forms twisting and contorting into nightmarish shapes that seemed to mock her attempts to cling to a sense of normalcy.

Amidst the storm of physical tics and haunting hallucinations, Sarah's family stood by her side, their love a beacon of light in the encroaching darkness. With each passing day, they witnessed the toll that these sinister visions took on their beloved daughter, their hearts heavy with a helplessness that threatened to consume them.

Yet, in the depths of despair, a glimmer of hope remained. Through the unwavering support of her family and the resilience that burned within her, Sarah found the strength to face the shadows that threatened to engulf her. With each step she took, each butterfly she chased, she forged a path towards acceptance, courage, and the unwavering belief that even in the darkest of moments, there existed a flicker of light waiting to guide her home.

As the manifestations of Sarah's condition intensified, her family sought solace and answers in the expertise of medical professionals. However, the once warm embrace of hope turned cold as the doctors, with furrowed brows and hesitant gazes, began to suggest that her symptoms might be rooted in a mental illness that defied easy categorization.

In the sterile confines of the clinic, the air hung heavy with unspoken doubts and unvoiced fears. The white-coated figures that surrounded Sarah spoke in hushed tones, their diagnoses cloaked in uncertainty and ambiguity. The once familiar faces now seemed distant, their expressions veiled behind a mask of clinical detachment that left her family reeling with a sense of abandonment.

As the words "psychiatric evaluation" and "mental health intervention" echoed through the sterile walls, a sense of isolation settled over Sarah like a suffocating shroud. The doctors, once beacons of knowledge and healing, now seemed unwilling to delve deeper into the labyrinth of her symptoms, their reluctance a barrier that stood between her and the help she so desperately sought.

Her family's pleas fell on deaf ears, their voices drowned out by the weight of medical opinion that deemed her condition beyond the realm of traditional treatment. The once vibrant hope that had buoyed their spirits now lay shattered at their feet, replaced by a sense of helplessness and despair that threatened to engulf them all.

Yet, amidst the bleak landscape of doubt and disregard, a flicker of defiance ignited within Sarah's soul. With a steely determination born of adversity, she refused to be defined by the limitations of others' perceptions. In the face of medical skepticism and professional reluctance, she clung to the belief that her truth was valid, her experiences real, and that within the depths of her being lay the resilience to rise above the shadows that sought to consume her.

Together with her unwavering family, Sarah embarked on a journey of self-discovery and empowerment, forging a path that defied conventional wisdom and embraced the complexities of her unique reality. In their united front against the tide of doubt and dismissal, they found a strength that transcended the confines of medical opinion, a bond that illuminated the darkness and paved the way towards a future where healing, understanding, and acceptance awaited.

When Sarah's tics escalated, they became unbearable. Her body moved uncontrollably, jerking her arms and legs in sudden, painful motions. The constant twitching made it hard for her to focus or even carry out daily tasks. Sarah's distress grew as her tics intensified, causing her physical pain and emotional strain. Desperate for relief, she sought help from a specialist to manage her condition and regain control over her body.

In the early hours of the morning, Sarah's tics took a frightening turn. What began as subtle twitches soon evolved into violent convulsions, akin to seizures. Her body contorted involuntarily, her muscles seizing up with alarming intensity. Despite her efforts to contain the movements, they only grew more pronounced and unmanageable.

As the minutes turned into hours, Sarah found herself trapped in a cycle of relentless spasms that left her exhausted and terrified. The once familiar tics now resembled a chaotic storm raging through her body, causing her immense pain and confusion.

In the last six hours, Sarah's world had been turned upside down by these unexpected seizures. Desperate for answers and relief, she knew she had to seek urgent medical attention to unravel this new and distressing chapter in her struggle with tics.

As Sarah continued to endure the distressing seizures, doctors were puzzled by the mystery underlying their cause. Despite a battery of tests and consultations with specialists, the medical team remained unable to pinpoint the origin of Sarah's escalating condition.

The uncertainty surrounding the seizures only added to Sarah's anxiety and frustration. She felt lost in a sea of unanswered questions, grappling with the fear of the unknown and the toll it was taking on her physical and emotional well-being. With each passing day, the enigma of her condition deepened, leaving her and her medical team grasping for a breakthrough that seemed just out of reach.

Feeling increasingly disillusioned and overwhelmed by the lack of progress in her treatment, Sarah was disheartened by the perceived ineffectiveness of the medical interventions thus far. The disconnect between her experiences and the doctors' inability to offer concrete solutions left her feeling stranded in a sea of uncertainty and vulnerability.

Despite the medical team's best efforts, the persistent absence of a definitive diagnosis or effective treatment plan only deepened Sarah's sense of frustration and helplessness. She longed for a beacon of hope, a glimmer of understanding that would illuminate the path towards relief and recovery. Yet, in the face of ongoing uncertainty, Sarah grappled with the daunting reality of navigating her health journey with scarce answers and diminishing faith in the medical system.

As Sarah grappled with the distressing reality of her unexplained seizures, the dismissive suggestion that her symptoms were merely "all in her head" added a new layer of frustration and disbelief to her already challenging journey. Despite her earnest attempts to seek validation and understanding from the medical professionals entrusted with her care, she found herself confronted with the disheartening implication that her struggles were being trivialized or misunderstood.

The notion that her symptoms were dismissed as psychological rather than physical further compounded Sarah's feelings of isolation and confusion. She yearned for a sense of validation and empathy that seemed elusive within the medical discourse surrounding her condition. As she navigated the complexities of her health struggles, Sarah found herself grappling not only with the burden of her symptoms but also with the weight of the stigma and skepticism that clouded her efforts to seek answers and support.

On a poignant Christmas Eve, Sarah's world was momentarily eclipsed by a distressing event that left her feeling vulnerable and isolated. As her left hand suddenly contorted in an agonizing cramp, seizing with an intensity that rendered it immobile and unresponsive, a wave of fear and helplessness washed over her. The stark contrast between the festive cheer enveloping her surroundings and the stark reality of her physical distress painted a poignant picture of her struggle.

In the quiet stillness of that fateful evening, Sarah's paralyzed hand served as a stark reminder of the unpredictability and cruelty of her condition. The inability to control her own body, coupled with the emotional weight of this somber occurrence on a day typically associated with joy and togetherness, cast a shadow over her festive spirit. In that moment of vulnerability and uncertainty, Sarah found herself grappling with a profound sense of disconnection and uncertainty, yearning for solace and understanding amidst the poignant backdrop of Christmas Eve.

As time passed, Sarah's journey took a harrowing turn as the temporary paralysis that once visited her left hand began to encroach upon her other limbs, each episode stretching into weeks of immobilizing confinement. The gradual escalation of her symptoms painted a chilling portrait of her escalating health crisis, as her body seemed to betray her with increasing frequency and intensity.

With each passing month, Sarah found herself grappling with the disheartening reality of her limbs succumbing to temporary paralysis, robbing her of mobility and autonomy for prolonged periods. The transient nature of these episodes added a layer of unpredictability and anxiety to her already tumultuous journey, leaving her in a state of perpetual unease and apprehension.

Navigating the challenges of daily life amid the specter of recurrent paralysis tested Sarah's resilience and fortitude, as she sought to maintain a semblance of normalcy in the face of this relentless onslaught on her physical well-being. The months that followed served as a stark reminder of the fragility of her health and the formidable obstacles she faced in her quest for answers and relief.

In a cruel twist of fate, Sarah's world was once again plunged into turmoil as a neurological stroke cast a shadow over her existence, leaving a trail of debilitating effects in its wake. The stroke's merciless assault on her nervous system manifested in a myriad of stark symptoms, each more profound and disorienting than the last.

The stroke's impact on Sarah's left eye was immediate and unforgiving, shrouding her world in a monochromatic veil of black and white, punctuated by a disorienting blur that distorted her perception of reality. The loss of color and clarity in her vision served as a stark reminder of the stroke's relentless grip on her senses, robbing her of the vibrant hues and intricate details that once defined her visual experience.

Furthermore, the stroke's insidious reach extended beyond her eyes, as Sarah found herself grappling with the profound loss of sensation and mobility in her left side. The paralysis that enveloped her left limbs rendered them inert and unresponsive, stripping away her ability to move and control a significant portion of her body. The absence of feeling in her left side further compounded her sense of disconnection from her own physical being, leaving her trapped in a state of immobilized vulnerability.

As Sarah navigated the daunting aftermath of her neurological stroke, she found herself confronted with a harsh new reality defined by limitations and challenges that tested her resilience and determination. The profound impact of the stroke on her senses, movement, and overall well-being served as a stark reminder of the fragility of life and the indomitable spirit required to navigate its darkest moments.

Just when it seemed that Sarah's struggles couldn't get any more daunting, a cruel twist of fate revealed a previously unknown allergy to Ativan, unleashing a cascade of additional challenges that further complicated her already tumultuous journey. The discovery of this adverse reaction to the medication cast a dark shadow over her treatment plan, setting off a chain reaction of distressing symptoms that plunged her into a nightmarish ordeal.

The allergic reaction to Ativan triggered a series of hallucinations that fractured Sarah's sense of reality, blurring the lines between the tangible and the imagined in a disorienting dance of vivid illusions and distorted perceptions. These hallucinations cast a surreal pall over her waking hours, infusing her everyday experiences with a sense of unreality and disconnection that eroded her sense of stability and security.

Moreover, the allergic response to Ativan also precipitated a deepening spiral of depression that enveloped Sarah in a suffocating fog of despair and despondency. The weight of this emotional burden bore down on her spirit, casting a long shadow over her mental well-being and exacerbating the already formidable challenges she faced in her battle for health and healing.

As Sarah's father sat vigilantly by her side in the sterile confines of the hospital room, his heart heavy with concern and his gaze filled with a mix of love and worry, he bore witness to a heart-wrenching scene that tugged at the very fabric of his being. The effects of the allergic reaction to Ativan had plunged Sarah into a realm of hallucinations so vivid and disorienting that they blurred the boundaries between reality and illusion, leaving her lost in a bewildering landscape of her mind's own making.

In the grip of these hallucinations, Sarah's perception of the world around her was distorted beyond recognition, as she watched in wonderment as imaginary children frolicked and played in the sterile corridors of the hospital, their laughter echoing through the empty spaces with a haunting melody that pierced the silence. Her father, a silent sentinel in this surreal tableau, could only watch helplessly as his daughter's mind danced to a tune only she could hear, a poignant reminder of the fragility of the human psyche in the face of adversity.

As the boundaries between the hospital room and the familiar comforts of home began to blur and fade, Sarah's confusion deepened, leading her to believe that she was in the comforting embrace of her own living room. The simple act of installing a bathroom in this newfound domestic space elicited a sense of wonder and gratitude in her altered state of mind, a testament to the disorienting power of the hallucinations that gripped her with an iron fist.

For Sarah's father, each moment spent by his daughter's side in the hospital was a poignant reminder of the tenuous nature of reality and the profound depths of love and sacrifice that defined their bond. As he bore witness to her struggles and triumphs, her moments of clarity and confusion, he drew strength from the unwavering resolve that burned bright in her eyes, a beacon of hope in the darkness that surrounded them.

In a stunning and disheartening turn of events, Sarah's neurologist delivered a chilling diagnosis that shattered the fragile veneer of hope that had sustained her in the midst of her trials. With a cold detachment that cut to the core of her being, the neurologist pronounced that the stroke, which Sarah had believed to be a tangible and harrowing reality, was nothing more than a figment of her imagination—a phantom affliction conjured by the recesses of her own mind.

For Sarah, this pronouncement was a devastating blow, a cruel twist of fate that undermined the very foundations of her sense of self and reality. To have her lived experience dismissed as mere delusion, to be told that the pain and suffering she endured were nothing more than a mirage, was a betrayal of the highest order—a betrayal of trust, of empathy, of the sacred bond between patient and healer.

As Sarah grappled with the crushing weight of this revelation, a storm raged within her, a tempest of conflicting emotions that threatened to consume her in its fiery embrace. Anger, confusion, disbelief, despair—all vied for dominance within her fractured psyche, each emotion a blade that cut deep into the tender fabric of her soul.

Yet, amidst the turmoil and chaos that engulfed her, a flicker of defiance sparked to life in Sarah's eyes—a flame of indomitable spirit that refused to be extinguished by the callous words of a dismissive physician. In that moment of reckoning, she vowed to rise above the doubts and denials that sought to erode her sense of self-worth, to forge a path forward guided by her own inner truth and resilience.

As Sarah stood on the precipice of uncertainty, her gaze fixed on the distant horizon of possibility, she knew that the road ahead would be fraught with challenges and obstacles, with doubters and naysayers lurking at every turn. But in the crucible of her own determination, she found the strength to defy the odds, to reclaim her agency, and to rewrite the narrative of her own healing journey on her own terms.

In a courageous and pivotal decision, Sarah and her family resolved to seek a second opinion from the esteemed pediatric specialists at the children's hospital—a beacon of hope and expertise in the realm of pediatric care. With hearts heavy with trepidation and hope intertwined, they embarked on a journey to unravel the mysteries that had plagued Sarah's health and well-being, to seek clarity and understanding in the face of uncertainty.

As they crossed the threshold of the children's hospital, a sense of anticipation and apprehension hung heavy in the air, mingling with the sterile scent of antiseptic and the soft hum of medical machinery. Yet, amidst the bustling corridors and hushed conversations that filled the space, there was a palpable sense of reassurance—a sense that they had entered a sanctuary of healing and compassion, a place where expertise and empathy converged to offer solace and solace in equal measure.

In the hallowed halls of the children's hospital, Sarah and her family were greeted by a team of dedicated specialists whose eyes shone with empathy and understanding, whose voices resonated with a sense of purpose and commitment to excellence. With meticulous attention to detail and unwavering dedication to their craft, the pediatric experts embarked on a thorough examination of Sarah's condition, leaving no stone unturned in their quest for answers and solutions.

As the days turned into weeks and the weeks into months, Sarah underwent a battery of tests and consultations, each one a stepping stone on the path to enlightenment and healing. The pediatric specialists worked tirelessly to unravel the complexities of Sarah's case, drawing on their collective expertise and experience to chart a course of action that held the promise of a brighter future for their young patient.

And in the end, as the dust settled and the echoes of uncertainty faded into the distance, Sarah and her family found themselves standing on the threshold of a new chapter in their lives—a chapter illuminated by the beacon of hope that had guided them through the darkest of times, a chapter defined by resilience, courage, and the unwavering belief in the power of healing and transformation.

In a moment of revelation and clarity, after several visits and consultations with the dedicated team of pediatric specialists at the children's hospital, a diagnosis finally emerged—an illuminating beacon of understanding that shed light on the complexities of Sarah's condition. The physiologists, armed with their expertise and compassion, identified the underlying cause of Sarah's struggles as Pediatric Acute-onset Neuropsychiatric Syndrome (PANS)—a diagnosis that brought both relief and a renewed sense of purpose to Sarah and her family.

With this diagnosis in hand, a roadmap to healing and recovery began to take shape—a roadmap that was tailored to Sarah's unique needs and challenges, to her individual journey towards well-being and wholeness. The physiologists, drawing on their deep well of knowledge and experience, crafted a comprehensive treatment plan that integrated medical interventions, therapy, and support systems designed to address the multifaceted dimensions of PANS and pave the way for Sarah's restoration to health.

As Sarah embarked on this transformative journey—a journey marked by setbacks and triumphs, by moments of doubt and resilience—she found herself surrounded by a dedicated team of caregivers and loved ones who stood by her side with unwavering commitment and unwavering faith. Together, they navigated the twists and turns of the healing process, drawing strength from each other and from the unwavering belief in Sarah's capacity to overcome adversity and emerge stronger on the other side.

With the skilled hands of healthcare professionals guiding the way, Sarah underwent the IVIG therapy sessions with courage and resilience, drawing strength from the unwavering support of her loved ones and the unwavering belief in the potential for healing and renewal. Each session marked a step towards progress, a step towards unlocking the doors of possibility and paving the way for a brighter future for Sarah and her family.

As the weeks unfolded and the effects of the IVIG treatment began to manifest, a sense of hope and gratitude washed over Sarah and her family—a sense that they were on the cusp of something extraordinary, something that held the promise of a new beginning and a brighter tomorrow. With each passing day, Sarah's journey towards healing gained momentum, fueled by the transformative power of IVIG and the unwavering belief in the resilience of the human spirit.

And in the end, as Sarah stood on the threshold of a new chapter in her life—a chapter defined by resilience, courage, and the unwavering belief in the power of healing and transformation—she knew in her heart that the IVIG treatment had been a turning point, a beacon of hope that had guided her through the darkest of times and illuminated the path towards a future filled with promise and possibility.

After undergoing three rounds of IVIG treatment, a remarkable transformation unfolded in Sarah's journey towards healing. The once-daunting shadows of her symptoms began to dissipate, giving way to the gentle glow of wellness and wholeness. With each treatment session, Sarah felt the tendrils of change weaving their magic, gradually lifting the veil of her illness and revealing the radiant light of her restored vitality.

As the effects of the IVIG treatment took hold, Sarah and her family witnessed a profound shift in her well-being—a shift marked by the gradual fading of her symptoms and the blossoming of hope and optimism in their hearts. The once-pervasive struggles that had defined Sarah's daily life began to recede, making room for a newfound sense of freedom and possibility.

With each passing day, Sarah embraced the joy of rediscovering the simple pleasures of life—the laughter of loved ones, the warmth of a sunlit day, the quiet beauty of a moment savored in tranquility. As her energy levels surged and her spirits lifted, Sarah felt a renewed sense of purpose and determination taking root within her, propelling her towards a future brimming with promise and potential.

And as the final round of IVIG treatment drew to a close, Sarah stood on the threshold of a new beginning—a beginning marked by resilience, courage, and the unwavering belief in the power of healing and transformation. Most of her symptoms had vanished, replaced by a sense of lightness and freedom that enveloped her like a gentle embrace, reminding her of the strength and resilience that had carried her through the darkest of times.

In the wake of the IVIG treatments, Sarah's journey towards wellness had blossomed into a testament to the indomitable spirit of the human heart—a spirit that had weathered the storms of adversity and emerged stronger, more radiant, and more alive than ever before. And as she looked towards the horizon of her future, Sarah knew with unwavering certainty that the path ahead was filled with endless possibilities, each one a testament to the power of hope, resilience, and the unwavering belief in the transformative power of healing.

Despite the profound improvements brought about by the IVIG treatment, Sarah understood that her journey towards wellness had its own unique trajectory. While she might not fully recover to her pre-illness state, she found solace and acceptance in the remnants of her tics that had become a part of her identity—a reminder of her resilience, her journey, and the strength that resided within her.

As Sarah reflected on her transformed life, she embraced the tics that lingered, recognizing them not as remnants of a past struggle, but as symbols of her journey and her unwavering spirit. These tics, once seen as adversaries, now stood as silent witnesses to her resilience, her courage, and the unwavering belief that had carried her through the darkest of times.

In a moment of introspection, Sarah realized that these remaining tics had woven themselves into the fabric of her being, becoming an integral part of her story and her identity. They were not blemishes to be erased, but rather threads that added depth and nuance to the tapestry of her life—a tapestry woven with moments of struggle, moments of triumph, and moments of quiet acceptance.

As she navigated the complexities of her post-treatment life, Sarah found comfort in the familiarity of these tics, a constant reminder of the battles she had fought and the victories she had won. They served as a beacon of resilience, a testament to her strength, and a source of grounding in a world that often seemed turbulent and uncertain.

Embracing the tics as a part of her being, Sarah found a sense of peace and acceptance—a recognition that they were not signs of weakness, but symbols of her unyielding spirit and her unwavering resolve. And as she moved forward on her journey, she carried with her the knowledge that these tics were not hindrances, but rather markers of her resilience, her courage, and the indomitable spirit that defined her very essence.

As Sarah embarked on her return to school, she carried with her the lessons of resilience, determination, and unwavering spirit that had defined her journey towards healing. With each step she took, she felt the echoes of her past struggles guiding her forward, propelling her towards new heights of achievement and success.

Supported by the unwavering love and assistance of her devoted sister, Sarah found herself navigating the challenges of academia with a newfound sense of purpose and clarity. Together, they formed an unbreakable bond—a bond forged in the fires of adversity and strengthened by the shared triumphs and trials that had shaped their lives.

As the school year unfolded, Sarah's academic prowess shone brightly, illuminating the path towards academic excellence and personal growth. With her sister by her side, she tackled each assignment, each exam, and each obstacle with grace, determination, and a deep sense of gratitude for the support and encouragement that surrounded her.

And as the final grades were tallied, Sarah stood side by side with her sister, both adorned with the mantle of high honors—a testament to their unwavering dedication, their unyielding spirit, and the profound bond that united them in their shared journey of triumph and transformation.

Together, they walked across the stage, their hearts brimming with pride and joy, as they accepted their well-deserved accolades and basked in the glow of their shared success. And in that moment, as the applause washed over them like a gentle wave, Sarah knew that she had not only conquered her struggles but had emerged victorious—a beacon of hope, strength, and resilience for all who witnessed her remarkable journey.

Despite the challenges of needing a walker to navigate and her legal blindness, Sarah's determination and unwavering passion for neurology fueled her incredible journey. Embracing her physical limitations as a testament to her resilience, she pursued her dream of becoming a neurologist specializing in Pediatric Acute-onset Neuropsychiatric Syndrome (PANS) with unparalleled dedication and fervor.

With the support of her colleagues, mentors, and assistive technology, Sarah overcame every obstacle that stood in her path. Her unique perspective as a patient with firsthand experience of neurological conditions enriched her approach to patient care and research, setting her apart in the field of neurology.

Through her unwavering commitment and expertise, Sarah emerged as a beacon of hope and inspiration for her patients, demonstrating that empathy, understanding, and a relentless pursuit of knowledge could transform lives and shape the future of medical practice.

As a pioneering neurologist specializing in PANS, she not only treated patients with compassion and skill but also conducted groundbreaking research that advanced the understanding and treatment of this complex syndrome. Sarah's journey from patient to healer exemplified the transformative power of resilience, determination, and unwavering dedication to a noble cause.

Her story inspired countless individuals facing similar challenges, showcasing that with perseverance, passion, and a steadfast belief in oneself, even the most formidable obstacles could be overcome. Sarah's legacy as a neurologist and advocate for patients with neurological conditions resonated far beyond the confines of a hospital or research lab, leaving an indelible mark on the field of medicine and the lives she touched.

In her role as a neurologist specializing in Pediatric Acute-onset Neuropsychiatric Syndrome (PANS), Sarah became a fierce advocate for children facing similar challenges. Drawing from her own experiences and struggles, she dedicated herself to ensuring that every child with PANS was heard, understood, and supported—not dismissed or told that their condition was "all in their head."

Through her tireless advocacy efforts, Sarah worked to raise awareness about PANS, educate healthcare professionals, and empower families to advocate for their children's needs. She spearheaded initiatives to promote early diagnosis, access to quality care, and comprehensive treatment options for children grappling with this complex neurological disorder.

By amplifying the voices of children with PANS, Sarah helped dismantle misconceptions and stigma surrounding the condition, fostering a more compassionate and inclusive healthcare system that prioritized listening to and valuing the experiences of young patients.

Her unwavering commitment to championing the rights and well-being of children with PANS not only transformed individual lives but also catalyzed systemic change within the medical community and beyond. Sarah's advocacy efforts served as a catalyst for a paradigm shift, ensuring that every child with PANS had a voice, a platform, and a champion in their corner.

Through her advocacy work, Sarah became a beacon of hope and empowerment, inspiring a new generation of healthcare providers, policymakers, and advocates to prioritize the needs and rights of children with neurological conditions. Her legacy as a compassionate healer, dedicated advocate, and tireless champion for children's voices continued to resonate, creating a brighter, more inclusive future for all those touched by PANS.

Amid life's challenges, Sarah held steadfast to her belief that everything happened for a reason. Despite the hardships she faced, Sarah found purpose and strength in her journey, understanding that her struggles had equipped her to address a profound need in the world.

Through her perseverance, resilience, and unwavering faith, Sarah emerged as a beacon of hope and healing for children with Pediatric Acute-onset Neuropsychiatric Syndrome (PANS). Her personal struggles had uniquely prepared her to empathize with and advocate for those facing similar challenges, guiding her towards a path of service and impact.

Sarah's unwavering trust in a greater plan fueled her determination to make a difference, reminding herself and others that even in the darkest moments, there was purpose and meaning waiting to be revealed. Her journey from adversity to advocacy exemplified the transformative power of faith, hope, and the unwavering belief in a brighter tomorrow.

As she embraced her calling to advocate for children with PANS, Sarah's past struggles took on new significance, shaping her into a compassionate healer and tireless champion for those in need. Through her work, she embodied the belief that every challenge carried within it the seeds of growth, resilience, and the potential to make a profound difference in the lives of others.

Sarah's story served as a testament to the transformative power of faith, perseverance, and a steadfast commitment to serving a greater purpose. In embracing her past struggles as stepping stones to a greater calling, she exemplified the resilience and grace that could emerge from life's most difficult trials.er six text here. Insert chapter six text here. Insert chapter six text here. Insert chapter six text here. Insert chapter six text here. Insert chapter six text here. Insert chapter six text here. Insert chapter six text here. Insert chapter six text here. Insert chapter six text here. Insert

ABOUT THE AUTHOR

I am not a writer in fact I failed English in High School. This is a story that is very true and words cannot describe how horrific the actual events were. I just want to bring awareness that affects way more children in the world then diagnosed. IF this story brings awareness and saves 1 child from torture, it will be a success.

In tough times, if you are saying "Why would God allow this to happen?" remember, he does it for a reason. Your struggle today, forms you into the person you become tomorrow. You too may just become a Neurologist with a purpose.